MAKING HERBAL SKIN CARE FOR BEGINNERS

Practical Knowledge Guide On Skills, Techniques And Pattern To Understand, Master & Explore The Process Of Herbal Skin Care Making From Scratch

HENRY HICKMAN

Disclaimer

The information provided in this book has been meticulously researched and compiled to ensure accuracy and completeness. However, it is important to note that the content within this book is intended solely for informational and educational purposes. It is not intended for self-prediction or as a guarantee of outcomes.

The author has dedicated considerable time and effort to present reliable information.

Nevertheless, the author cannot be held responsible for any potential omission of words or content within this book.

Furthermore, the author hereby declares no affiliation or agreement with any website, individual, product or platform in the form of affiliate or any other kind. This book is created purely for educational purposes.

Readers are advised that the author will not be liable for any loss or consequences, whether direct or indirect, arising from the use or misuse of the information contained in this book. It is recommended to exercise discretion and consult additional sources or professionals when implementing the techniques or information provided herein.

By using this book, readers agree to do so at their own discretion and assume full responsibility for any actions taken based on the content presented.

Table of Contents

CHAPTER 1

Introduction

Herbal skin care entails harnessing the power of nature to improve the skin's health and look. This holistic skincare technique incorporates the use of numerous plants recognized for their medicinal characteristics.

Unlike commercial skincare products, which can include synthetic components, herbal skincare emphasizes natural therapies that have been utilized in traditional medicine for generations. Herbal skincare production is a fascinating journey that blends old wisdom with contemporary expertise, from choosing the perfect herbs to understanding their qualities and extraction and processing procedures.

Understanding Herbal Ingredients

The careful selection of plants is the core of herbal skincare. Different herbs have different skin advantages, and their efficacy might vary depending on variables such as skin type and particular skin conditions.

Aloe vera, chamomile, calendula, lavender, and rosemary are all popular skincare herbs. Each herb brings something special to the table, such as anti-inflammatory, antibacterial, or hydrating characteristics. The combination of these herbs results in a strong formulation that tackles a variety of skin concerns while supporting a natural and gentle approach to skincare.

Selection Of Herbs

The selection of plants is an important stage in the production of herbal skincare. Understanding the individual demands of various skin types and conditions is critical for selecting the proper herb combination. Chamomile, for example, is well-known for its calming effects, making it ideal for sensitive or irritated skin. Herbs like rosemary and tea tree oil, on the other hand, are regarded for their antibacterial and antiseptic properties, making them good for acne-prone skin. The specific qualities of each plant are carefully considered to provide a well-balanced and effective herbal skin care composition.

Properties Of Herbs For Skin Care

Herbs have a variety of characteristics that may help the skin in a variety of ways. Some herbs are high in antioxidants, which aid in the fight against free radicals, which lead to premature aging. Others contain anti-inflammatory characteristics that help soothe and diminish redness in sensitive skin. Many plants include vitamins and minerals that help to nourish and revitalize the skin.

For example, vitamin C in plants like rosehip may boost collagen formation, which helps with skin suppleness. Understanding these qualities enables skincare aficionados to build solutions that treat particular skin disorders while also promoting general skin health.

Extracting And Processing Herbs

Following the selection of the plants, the beneficial chemicals are extracted. Infusions, maceration, and distillation are common extraction processes. Infusions include steeping plants in a carrier oil to progressively extract their qualities.

Maceration is the process of soaking herbs in oil for a lengthy period to allow for more effective extraction. Distillation, which is often used for essential oils, involves passing steam through plants to capture aromatic and medicinal ingredients.

The herbal extracts are meticulously processed after extraction into different skincare products such as creams, serums, and toners. Proper processing preserves the potency of the herbs while producing products that are safe and stable for usage.

To summarize, herbal skincare production is a comprehensive and sophisticated process that requires a thorough study of plants, their qualities, and the skill of extraction. This method not only solves many skin issues but also links people with nature's healing power. By adopting herbal skincare, one may begin on a road to healthier, more vibrant skin while also appreciating the knowledge handed down through centuries in the use of natural medicines.

CHAPTER 2

Essential Oils In Herbal Skin Care

Herbal skincare enhanced with essential oils has grown in popularity as a holistic approach to skin nurturing and revitalization. Essential oils, which are concentrated extracts of plants, play an important part in the formulation of natural skincare products. These oils are valued in herbal skincare compositions not only for their fragrant characteristics but also for their therapeutic advantages. Essential oils, ranging from lavender to tea tree, are an important step in creating effective and safe herbal skincare solutions.

Choosing The Right Essential Oils

The creation of herbal skincare starts with the careful selection of essential oils. Each essential oil has distinct qualities that cater to certain skincare requirements.

Lavender oil, for example, is well-known for its relaxing and soothing properties, making it great for sensitive or irritated skin. Tea tree oil, on the other hand, is known for its antibacterial characteristics, making it a popular treatment for acne and blemishes. Understanding the unique properties of essential oils enables skincare aficionados and formulators to personalize their products to specific skin types and issues. When selecting an herbal skincare mix, it is important to examine elements such as the oil's extraction technique, purity, and compatibility with other oils.

Benefits Of Essential Oils For The Skin

The advantages of essential oils in herbal skincare are many and go beyond simply smell. These oils are high in antioxidants, vitamins, and fatty acids, which help to improve skin health and attractiveness.

Essential oils include antioxidants that help fight free radicals, avoiding premature aging and maintaining young skin. Furthermore, essential oils have anti-inflammatory and antibacterial qualities, making them useful in the treatment of skin disorders such as acne, eczema, and psoriasis. Certain oils' hydrating properties make them good complements to herbal healthcare, treating dryness and increasing skin suppleness. Using essential oils for therapeutic purposes provides a well-rounded and holistic approach to skincare that addresses both the physical and emotional elements of well-being.

Blending Essential Oils Safely

While essential oils have several advantages, it is important to approach mixing with caution. These concentrated extracts may be very concentrated, and poor mixing might cause skin irritation or unpleasant reactions.

Dilution is an important safety precaution that ensures essential oils are combined with carrier oils or other acceptable bases to diminish their potency. Understanding the correct dilution ratios for each essential oil is critical in producing formulas that are effective while also being gentle on the skin. Patch testing is another important step in identifying any sensitivities or allergies before broad use. Furthermore, taking into account the synergy between various essential oils improves the overall effectiveness of the combination. Combining complementary oils not only optimizes their respective effects but also produces a harmonic and appealing scent. Overall, safe essential oil mixing is an art that requires a careful balance of creativity and adherence to the best standards, resulting in a skincare product that is not only effective but also mild and well-tolerated by the skin.

CHAPTER 3

Base Ingredients For Herbal Skin Care

Herbal skin care is gaining popularity due to its natural and holistic approach to skin health promotion. The cornerstone of any herbal skin care product is its basic components, which comprise the formulation's core structure.

substances have been chosen for their nourishing, hydrating, and therapeutic effects. The basic ingredients serve as a solid foundation for the incorporation of numerous plant extracts, essential oils, and other active substances that increase the therapeutic advantages of the finished product.

Carrier Oils And Their Properties

Carrier oils are the principal vehicle for delivering herbal extracts and essential oils to the skin in herbal skin care products.

These oils are high in fatty acids, vitamins, and antioxidants and are extracted from seeds, nuts, or fruits. Jojoba oil, for example, closely mimics the skin's natural sebum, making it an effective moisturizer for all skin types. Because of its lightweight texture and high vitamin E concentration, sweet almond oil is ideal for relaxing and nourishing the skin. Each carrier oil has a distinct set of qualities that enable formulators to adapt solutions to individual skin demands.

Butters And Waxes

Butter and waxes are important ingredients in herbal skin care formulations because they contribute to the texture, thickness, and general consistency of the products.

Shea butter, produced from shea tree nuts, is a popular option because of its creamy texture and deep moisturizing qualities.

Cocoa butter is recognized for its skin-nourishing and softening effects, as well as its chocolaty scent. Another frequent component is beeswax, which acts as a natural barrier on the skin, helping to seal in moisture and protect against external irritants. These butter and waxes not only improve the feel of the product but also give extra skin benefits.

Other Base Ingredients

Herbal skin care formulations may use various basic components in addition to carrier oils, butter, and waxes to improve effectiveness and attractiveness.

Aloe vera gel, for example, is well-known for its soothing and moisturizing characteristics, making it a popular ingredient in treatments for sensitive or sun-damaged skin. Glycerin is a humectant, which draws moisture to the skin and promotes hydration.

Clays like kaolin and bentonite may be used to give mild exfoliation and detoxification. Because of these numerous basic components, formulators may build a broad variety of herbal skin care solutions that are suited to specific skin issues.

Finally, knowing the significance of basic components is critical in creating successful herbal skin care formulations. Carrier oils, butter, and waxes serve as the base, while other components offer distinctive qualities to the finished product. The combination of these components not only maintains the stability and texture of the product but also increases the therapeutic advantages for healthier, more radiant skin.

CHAPTER 4

Basic Tools And Equipment

Herbal skin care products are created by combining science and nature, with a focus on using plant-based substances to improve skin health. To begin this journey, one must first get acquainted with the fundamental tools and equipment required for creating these natural compositions.

Mixing Utensils

Any herbal skin care formulation relies on mixing equipment. These include spatulas, spoons, and whisks, which should preferably be constructed of non-reactive materials like glass or stainless steel.

The selection of utensils is critical to prevent chemical interactions with herbal substances while keeping their potency and usefulness.

Furthermore, having a variety of sizes and shapes guarantees that variable amounts and consistencies of components may be accommodated throughout the formulation process. Cleaning and maintaining these tools properly is critical to preventing contamination and ensuring the purity of the end product.

Storage Containers

Once the herbal skin care products are created, they must be properly stored to retain their integrity over time. To protect the formulations from light, which might deteriorate some herbal constituents, dark glass or opaque plastic containers are often recommended.

Airtight containers assist in keeping things fresh and effective by preventing air exposure. It's a good idea to have a choice of container sizes to accommodate varying batch sizes. Labeling is also essential for keeping track of components, formulation dates, and expiry dates. Proper storage not only increases product shelf life but also improves the overall quality of herbal skin care items.

Safety Precautions

When producing herbal skin care, it is important to ensure safety. This entails adopting safety measures throughout the formulation process. Wearing protective equipment, such as gloves and a lab coat, reduces the chance of skin irritation or allergic responses to some herbal compounds.

Workplace ventilation is critical to avoid inhaling any airborne particles or pollutants. Furthermore, a fundamental grasp of each herb's qualities is essential to minimize any allergic responses or harmful consequences. Adherence to dosing standards and handling practices assures that herbal skin care products are not only effective but also safe to use.

Finally, mastering the skill of preparing herbal skin care requires a careful selection of mixing instruments, adequate storage containers, and rigorous attention to safety procedures. These aspects work together to provide high-quality, natural skin care products that harness the advantages of herbs while emphasizing the well-being of both the formulator and the end-user.

CHAPTER 5

Making Herbal Infusions And Extracts

Herbal skin care products are created by combining the healing and rejuvenating qualities of several herbs to produce natural and effective treatments. Making herbal infusions and extracts is an important part of this procedure. Herbal infusions and extracts are effective methods to include herbal medicinal properties in cosmetics products. Let's look at each one separately:

Infusing Oils With Herbs

Infusing oils with herbs is a time-honored process of extracting therapeutic chemicals from plants that have been utilized for generations. This method includes steeping dried herbs or plant components in a carrier oil for an extended period. Olive oil, jojoba oil, and sweet almond oil are common carrier oils for herbal infusions.

The selection of herbs is determined by the desired attributes; for example, chamomile is recognized for its calming benefits, whilst calendula is regarded for its skin-healing capabilities. The infusion process enables the oil to absorb the active ingredients of the herbs, resulting in a strong basis for lotions, balms, and salves.

Creating Herbal Extracts

Herbal extracts are concentrated solutions that capture the essence of the therapeutic characteristics of a plant. They may be created using a variety of solvents, including alcohol, glycerin, and vinegar.

Breaking down the plant material to liberate its active chemicals is part of the extraction process. Because alcohol easily extracts both water-soluble and fat-soluble plant elements, alcohol-based extracts, known as tinctures, are very popular in herbal skincare formulations. Lavender, rosemary, and green tea are some of the most widely utilized herbs for extracts. Herbal extracts provide antioxidants, anti-inflammatory agents, and other healing characteristics to skincare products.

Using Infusions In Skin Care Recipes

Herbal infusions and extracts may be readily included in a variety of skincare formulas once prepared. These plant compounds improve the effectiveness of skincare formulas, providing a natural alternative to synthetically loaded commercially available treatments.

An herbal-infused oil, for example, might be a major element in a moisturizing lotion or face serum, offering nutrition while also supporting skin health. Herbal extracts may be used as toners, masks, or creams to provide specialized advantages such as anti-aging, acne-fighting, or skin-calming properties. Herbal infusions and extracts' adaptability enables formulators to personalize their skincare products to target particular skin conditions, making them an important component of natural skincare.

Finally, the skill of creating herbal skincare products entails the careful incorporation of herbal infusions and extracts. Skincare aficionados may leverage the healing qualities of plants by infusing oils with herbs and making strong extracts. These plant elements, which are high in vitamins, antioxidants, and other bioactive substances, may then be used in a variety of skincare regimens to achieve healthy and glowing skin.

CHAPTER 6

Creating Herbal Skin Care Products

Herbal Face Masks

Herbal face masks have become quite popular in the world of natural skincare. These masks often include herbs recognized for their skin-nourishing effects. Turmeric, neem, aloe vera, and chamomile may be used to make masks that target certain skin conditions.

Turmeric, for example, has anti-inflammatory and brightening effects, whilst aloe vera soothes and moisturizes the skin. The herbs are ground or blended into a fine powder, which is then combined with a base, such as yogurt or honey, to produce a paste. This paste is applied to the face and kept on for a certain amount of time to enable the herbal combination to permeate the skin and deliver medicinal advantages.

Herbal Toners And Mists

Herbal toners and mists are invigorating and refreshing complements to any skincare regimen. These products are generally liquids infused with herbal extracts or hydrosols obtained by the steam distillation of plant material.

Toners often include herbs such as rosemary, lavender, and witch hazel. Rosemary, for example, has astringent characteristics, whilst lavender has a relaxing effect.

To make an herbal toner, soak dried herbs in a liquid base, such as distilled water or witch hazel, and let the combination infuse.

The resultant liquid may be sprayed or applied to the skin with a cotton pad for a mild but efficient technique to tone and moisturize it.

Herbal Salves And Balms

Herbal salves and balms are concentrated compositions that are intended to treat particular skin ailments or to give deep nutrition. Herbs having therapeutic characteristics, such as calendula, comfreys, and lavender, are often included in these products.

Calendula is a common ingredient in salves because of its anti-inflammatory and skin-soothing properties. Dried herbs are infused in a carrier oil, such as olive or coconut oil, over time to make these formulations.

This infused oil is then combined with beeswax to form a salve or balm. The finished solution may be used topically to treat dry skin, small wounds, and irritation, making it a flexible and natural alternative to conventional ointments.

Herbal Scrubs And Cleansers

Herbal scrubs and cleansers exfoliate and wash the skin in a gentle but effective manner. These products often include exfoliating herbs like oats, pulverized almonds, or herbal powders like hibiscus.

To make a scrub or cleanser, the herbs are blended with a base such as honey, yogurt, or aloe vera gel. The abrasive granules exfoliate the skin, while the herbal compounds give extra advantages.

Hibiscus, for example, is high in antioxidants and may help you seem younger. The use of herbal scrubs and cleansers regularly helps to unclog pores, improve skin texture, and increase skin shine.

Herbal Moisturizers

Herbal moisturizers use a combination of herbs and natural oils to hydrate and nourish the skin. Shea butter, coconut oil, and herbal infusions like chamomile or rosehip are often utilized.

These natural oils and herbs were selected for their ability to seal in moisture and nourish the skin. Blending these components to obtain a creamy consistency is required for making herbal moisturizers.

The finished product may be used on both the face and the body to provide a rich and luxurious treatment that leaves the skin smooth and supple. Furthermore, the herbs utilized in these formulas often contain antioxidants and vitamins, providing an additional layer of defense against environmental stresses.

Finally, creating herbal skincare products entails using the therapeutic and nourishing characteristics of numerous plants. Each product category, from face masks to moisturizers, provides a distinct approach to improving skin health. Herbal skincare offers a holistic and natural alternative to conventional cosmetics, appealing to people wanting a greater connection to nature in their beauty regimens, whether treating particular ailments or boosting general well-being.

CHAPTER 7

Tailoring Products For Different Skin Types

Oily Skin

To create herbal skincare solutions for oily skin, substances that help manage excess oil production without depleting the skin of its natural moisture must be used. Oily skin benefits from herbs such as witch hazel, neem, and aloe vera. These substances have astringent characteristics that may aid in the tightening of pores and the regulation of oil secretion.

To prevent acne and pimples, an herbal cleanser for oily skin can include tea tree oil, which is recognized for its antimicrobial characteristics. Hydration may be provided by lightweight herbal moisturizers containing non-comedogenic oils such as jojoba or grapeseed.

Dry Skin

To address dryness and flakiness, herbal skincare for dry skin focuses on nourishing and moisturizing components. Herbs with calming and hydrating characteristics, such as calendula, chamomile, and lavender, are wonderful selections.

To preserve and promote moisture, an herbal cleanser for dry skin may include substances such as honey or olive oil. Herbal moisturizers including shea butter, coconut oil, or almond oil may provide the vital fats and moisture that dry skin needs. Incorporating anti-inflammatory herbs helps to soothe any discomfort caused by dryness.

Sensitive Skin

To prevent irritation and redness, sensitive skin demands delicate and calming herbal components. Because of its relaxing characteristics, chamomile, calendula, and aloe vera are popular options.

To wash without irritating, an herbal cleanser for sensitive skin might be prepared with chamomile tea or cucumber extract. Herbal moisturizers with few ingredients and no harsh chemicals may give the moisture that sensitive skin needs. Avoiding possible irritants like scents and utilizing anti-inflammatory herbs helps keep sensitive skin in check.

Combination Skin

Combination skin requires a balanced strategy that addresses both oily and dry regions. Ingredients in herbal skincare products for combination skin may include rosemary, green tea, and aloe vera. A moderate exfoliator, like oatmeal, may be used in an herbal cleanser for combination skin to handle both dry and oily areas. Lightweight herbal moisturizers with a combination of moisturizing and astringent herbs may aid in skin balance. Herbal toners containing components such as rose water may help tone and soothe both oily and dry areas of the skin, encouraging overall skin harmony.

To summarize, adapting herbal skincare solutions to various skin types entails choosing particular herbs and components that satisfy each skin type's distinct demands. Astringent and antibacterial herbs improve oily skin while nourishing and hydrating substances benefit dry skin. Sensitive skin needs mild, soothing herbs, and combination skin requires a balanced treatment that treats both dry and oily regions.

CHAPTER 8

Addressing Common Skin Issues

Acne And Blemishes

Herbal skincare formulas have grown in popularity due to their effectiveness in treating common skin concerns, including acne and pimples. Herbs like tea tree oil, neem, and aloe vera may be used in skin care products to give a natural and mild remedy for acne-prone skin. These herbs have antibacterial characteristics that aid in the fight against acne-causing bacteria, while aloe vera soothes and lowers irritation. Herbal components like chamomile and calendula may also be incorporated for their relaxing properties, which promote general skin health and assist in the decrease of blemishes.

Aging Skin

Herbal skincare takes a comprehensive approach to fighting the effects of aging by feeding the skin from the inside. Rosehip oil, which is high in vitamin C, contributes to collagen formation, enhancing skin suppleness, and minimizing the appearance of fine lines and wrinkles. Green tea extract and ginseng, for example, are herbal antioxidants that protect the skin from free radicals, preventing premature aging. Incorporating these herbs into face serums or creams may have a renewing impact, encouraging a younger and more luminous complexion.

Sun Damage

Sun protection is essential for preserving healthy and youthful-looking skin. Anti-inflammatory characteristics of herbal substances such as lavender oil and calendula extract help soothe burnt skin and assist in the healing process. Including herbs with natural SPF characteristics in skincare formulas, such as red raspberry seed oil and carrot seed oil, may give an extra layer of protection against dangerous UV radiation. Herbal sunscreens provide a chemical-free option for people who have sensitive skin or want a more natural approach to sun protection.

Eczema And Psoriasis

Skin disorders such as eczema and psoriasis need mild and nourishing skincare products. Chamomile, calendula, and lavender are herbal medicines that may help soothe inflamed skin, decrease inflammation, and relieve itching. Incorporating anti-inflammatory herbs into lotions or balms, such as chamomile, may give relief to eczema-prone skin. Herbal elements like aloe vera and burdock root may be good for psoriasis because of their hydrating and anti-inflammatory characteristics, which aid in calming the skin and minimizing flare-ups. These herbal treatments are excellent for those with sensitive skin since they are mild and natural.

Finally, herbal skincare products provide a natural and holistic approach to treating common skin concerns. It is possible to produce effective remedies for acne, aging skin, sun damage, and skin disorders such as eczema and psoriasis by knowing the qualities of certain herbs and putting them into skincare products. Herbal components' adaptability enables the creation of tailored skincare regimens that respond to specific skin demands, producing a healthier and more vibrant complexion.

Herbal Skin Care For Specific Needs

Herbal skin care has grown in popularity due to its natural and holistic approach to skin health. One of the most intriguing parts of herbal skin care is its capacity to address individual requirements. Herbal treatments provide a broad and effective variety of options, whether it's addressing the special issues of pregnant and postpartum skin, adapting formulations for men's skin, or guaranteeing the sensitive care of children's skin.

Pregnancy And Postpartum Skin Care

Pregnancy and postpartum periods cause major changes in a woman's body, particularly her skin. During this period, frequent concerns include hormonal swings, stretch marks, and heightened sensitivity.

Herbal skin care during pregnancy and postpartum focuses on giving treatments that are gentle, nutritious, and safe. Chamomile, calendula, and lavender are often used for their calming effects, while oils like almond and jojoba aid with moisture. To guarantee the health of both the mother and the newborn, formulations should emphasize the avoidance of harsh chemicals and allergies.

Men's Herbal Skin Care

Men's skin is different from women's, and herbal skin care understands and responds to these distinctions. Men often have thicker skin, wider pores, and a greater proclivity for oiliness. Herbal skin care for men usually contains substances that satisfy these unique requirements. Tea tree oil, for example, is recognized for its antibacterial characteristics, making it useful for acne management and reducing ingrown hairs.

Aloe vera and chamomile are calming ingredients that may help relieve post-shave discomfort. Herbal elements not only nourish the skin, but they also correspond with the growing interest in sustainable and natural grooming techniques.

Herbal Skin Care For Children

The skin of children is sensitive and needs extra care to retain its natural balance. Herbal skin care for children emphasizes the use of mild, hypoallergenic, and chemical-free components. Calendula, recognized for its soothing characteristics, is widely included in diaper rash and other skin irritation creams and lotions.

Bath products containing lavender and chamomile may encourage relaxation and assist in sleep. The focus is on simplicity and safety, with the products being devoid of any dangerous ingredients that may be absorbed via the skin.

Finally, herbal skincare that is adapted to particular requirements demonstrates a conscientious and sensitive approach to general well-being. Herbal treatments provide a perfect combination of nature and science to nourish and protect the skin, whether it's the specific difficulties of pregnancy, the different qualities of men's skin, or the gentle care necessary for infants. Herbal skin care's holistic concept corresponds with the rising inclination for sustainable and natural solutions, making it a flexible and attractive alternative for people at all stages of life.

CHAPTER 10

Tips For Formulating Your Own Recipes

Making herbal skin care is a fascinating and satisfying effort that enables people to develop bespoke skincare solutions that are matched to their specific requirements. Making your herbal skincare recipes involves a thorough awareness of many factors, including ratios, ingredients, experimentation, documentation, and modification. By diving into these fundamental ideas, one may realize the full potential of herbal components and harness their therapeutic effects for optimum skin health.

Understanding Ratios

Ratios are important in the creation of herbal skincare products. It entails measuring components precisely to achieve a balanced and effective result. Each component adds to the formulation's overall synergy by affecting its texture, absorption, and medicinal qualities. For example, the water-to-oil ratio in a formulation might affect the product's consistency and hydration levels. A thorough grasp of ratios contributes to product stability and effectiveness. Formulators may fine-tune their recipes by experimenting with various ratios to get the desired texture and performance.

Experimenting With Ingredients

Herbal skincare has a wide range of botanicals, oils, extracts, and other natural components, each with its own set of skin advantages. Experimentation is essential to find the ideal blend that treats certain skin conditions. Formulators may experiment with a broad variety of herbs renowned for anti-inflammatory, antioxidant, or moisturizing effects.

Carrier oils like jojoba, coconut, or argan oil may also be blended with herbal infusions to make nutritious mixtures. Experimentation may be used to discover the synergistic effects of several components, resulting in formulations that cater to certain skin types and problems.

Documenting And Adjusting

Accurate documentation is essential in the production of herbal skincare. Formulators can repeat successful formulas and fix any difficulties that may develop by keeping precise records of the materials used, their relative amounts, and the production process.

It is critical to record not just the chemicals but also the sensory properties and observable skin effects. This material will be useful for future formulations and changes. Formulators may tweak their formulas based on customer feedback and personal observations by examining and analyzing these data regularly, assuring continual progress and the production of successful skincare products.

To summarize, creating herbal skincare is a dynamic process that involves a thorough grasp of ratios, components, testing, documentation, and modification. Individuals may go on a creative adventure to develop bespoke skincare solutions that harness the power of nature for healthy and glowing skin by learning these ideas. Making herbal skincare, whether a relaxing face serum, a renewing mask, or a delicious body butter, provides limitless opportunities for self-expression and self-care.

CHAPTER 11

Packaging And Storing Herbal Skin Care Products

The packaging and storage of herbal skin care products are crucial to preserving their effectiveness and assuring user safety. Each step, from selecting the proper containers to labeling and date, is critical to protecting the purity of these natural compositions. Furthermore, knowing shelf life factors is critical for both manufacturers and customers to make educated product consumption and storage choices.

Choosing The Right Containers

Choosing the right container for herbal skin care products is critical to preserving the formulation's integrity. Dark glass or opaque plastic containers are often selected because they shield the contents from light, which may diminish the efficacy of herbal substances. When exposed to sunlight, light-sensitive chemicals in herbs, such as antioxidants, may degrade. Furthermore, airtight containers assist in preventing the introduction of air and moisture, which might undermine the product's stability. It is also critical to use containers made of materials that will not interact with the herbal extracts or essential oils to retain the product's purity.

Labeling And Dating

Herbal skin care products need clear and precise labeling. A detailed label should contain a list of contents, directions for use, and any dangers or contraindications.

Proper product labeling enables customers to make educated decisions based on their specific skin requirements and possible sensitivities. Furthermore, a production and expiry date are required for quality control and customer safety.

This data assists consumers in understanding the product's chronology and when it is most effective. It also assists manufacturers with inventory management and ensuring that only fresh items reach the market.

Shelf Life Considerations

Both producers and customers need to understand the shelf life of herbal skin care products. Natural goods, although frequently devoid of preservatives, may nonetheless be contaminated by microbes.

Shelf life may be affected by factors such as the kind of preservatives employed, storage conditions, and the quantity of water in formulations. Manufacturers must do stability testing to assess how long their goods will be effective and safe. On the consumer side, knowing a product's shelf life allows them to utilize it within the prescribed time frame, assuring optimum benefits and lowering the chance of unwanted reactions. Furthermore, careful storage, such as keeping items out of direct sunlight and severe temperatures, may help to extend their shelf life.

Finally, packing and storing herbal skin care products need close attention to detail. The selection of containers, labeling methods, and shelf life considerations all contribute to the overall quality and safety of these natural formulations. Understanding and executing these principles is critical to the success of herbal skin care, whether you are a manufacturer looking to preserve product purity or a customer looking for the greatest outcomes.

CHAPTER 12

Marketing And Selling Herbal Skin Care Products

Marketing and selling herbal skin care products requires a holistic strategy that takes into account both the specific elements of herbal formulations as well as the dynamics of the skincare industry. Herbal skincare products often appeal to people looking for natural alternatives, underscoring the need to promote organic and plant-based components in marketing efforts.

It is critical to educate people about the advantages of these herbs in skincare, demonstrating their usefulness in nourishing and rejuvenating the skin. Collaborations with celebrities and skincare professionals who can attest to the effectiveness of herbal substances might be part of marketing initiatives. It is critical to transmit a holistic message, highlighting not just the skincare advantages of herbal medicines, but also the general well-being connected with their use.

Compliance And Regulations

Compliance with laws is critical in the herbal skincare sector. The legal environment for cosmetics differs from country to country, and knowing the unique regulations for herbal products is critical.

This includes thorough ingredient testing, safety evaluations, and labeling regulations adherence. Compliance with rules fosters customer confidence by ensuring the quality and safety of the items.

Furthermore, being open about the source and manufacturing procedures of herbal substances might boost trust. Staying up to speed on regulatory changes is a continual obligation that must be met to alter formulations and marketing materials and ensure that the goods match the most recent standards and criteria.

Branding And Packaging

Branding is critical in distinguishing herbal skincare goods in a crowded market. It is critical to create a brand identity that captures the spirit of natural and herbal ingredients.

This includes creating a visually attractive logo, using earthy and organic color palettes, and creating a brand story that stresses the relationship between nature and skincare. Packaging is also important since it is the consumer's initial point of contact.

Sustainable and eco-friendly packaging not only complements the herbal theme but also speaks to the growing desire for ecologically conscientious options.

The packaging should convey the brand's devotion to purity and natural components, producing a captivating visual tale that entices prospective buyers.

Conclusion

Embracing Herbal Skin Care

Using herbal skincare is more than just a fad; it is a comprehensive approach to self-care that emphasizes the health of both the skin and the body. The move to herbal skincare is a deliberate decision to choose nature's abundance over manufactured and possibly dangerous chemicals. Individuals who use herbal alternatives actively contribute to sustainable practices and lessen their environmental imprint. Herbal skincare's nourishing and therapeutic properties go beyond just cosmetic improvements, establishing a deeper connection with the natural world.

Continuing Your Herbal Journey

Herbal skincare is a continual research of plant variety and the infinite possibilities it provides. Individuals' desire to develop this relationship deepens as they observe the wonderful benefits of herbal formulations on their skin. Experimenting with new herbs, perfecting recipes, and gaining knowledge about the vast world of plant-based skincare is all part of continuing the herbal journey.

It also fosters a feeling of empowerment by teaching folks how to design items that are personalized to their requirements. The herbal journey is a dynamic and ever-changing process that fosters a deep appreciation for the natural treasures that contribute to healthy, vibrant skin. As the trip progresses, so does the realization that herbal skincare is more than simply a regimen, but a way of life that aligns with the natural cycles.

THE END